Coronary Heart Disease Solution Guide

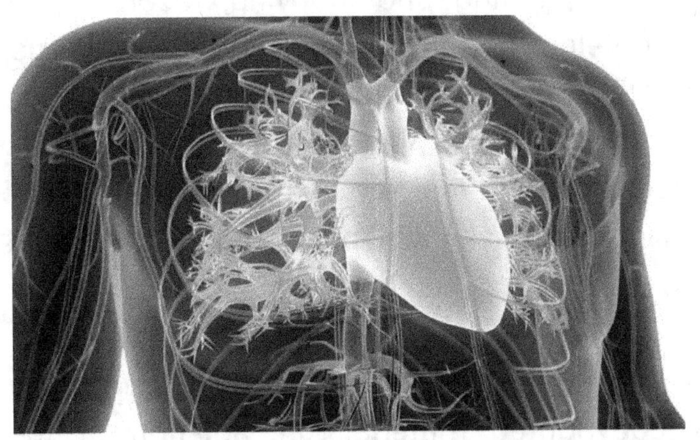

The Complete Step by Step Guide for Effective Diagnosis, Treatment, Prevention and Management

Dr Elizabeth Williams

Table of Contents

Forward

In the journey of healthcare, knowledge is our most powerful tool. As we navigate the complex landscape of coronary heart disease, it is imperative to arm ourselves with understanding, empathy, and a commitment to holistic care. It is with great pleasure that I introduce this invaluable guide on coronary heart disease.

Coronary heart disease stands as a formidable challenge in the realm of cardiovascular health, affecting millions worldwide and exerting a profound impact on individuals, families, and communities. Its multifaceted nature demands a multifaceted approach—one that encompasses not only medical interventions but also lifestyle modifications, emotional support, and patient education.

This guide represents a beacon of enlightenment in the realm of cardiovascular care.

Authored by esteemed cardiologists and healthcare professionals, it distills years of clinical expertise, research findings, and patient insights into a comprehensive roadmap for understanding, managing, and ultimately triumphing over coronary heart disease.

From the elucidation of pathophysiological mechanisms to the elucidation of treatment modalities, each chapter serves as a testament to the collective efforts of dedicated individuals committed to advancing the frontiers of cardiovascular medicine. But beyond the realms of science and technology, this guide delves into the human aspect of coronary heart disease—the fears, the uncertainties, and the triumphs that define the patient experience.

As you embark on this journey, may you find solace in the knowledge that you are not alone. Whether you are a patient grappling with the challenges of diagnosis, a caregiver offering unwavering support, or a healthcare professional advocating for optimal patient care, let this guide serve as a steadfast companion—a beacon of hope in times of uncertainty.

In closing, I extend my heartfelt gratitude to the authors, contributors, and healthcare professionals whose tireless dedication has brought this guide to fruition. May it illuminate the path toward better cardiovascular health, empower individuals to make informed decisions, and inspire a collective commitment to combating coronary heart disease with courage, compassion, and resilience.

Preface

Welcome to the comprehensive guide on coronary heart disease. As a cardiologist, I've encountered countless individuals grappling with the complexities of this condition, each with their unique concerns and questions. This guide aims to provide a thorough understanding of coronary heart disease, offering insights into its causes, symptoms, diagnosis, treatment options, and beyond.

Coronary heart disease is a formidable adversary, affecting millions worldwide and presenting formidable challenges to both patients and healthcare professionals. Its impact extends far beyond the physical realm, touching upon emotional, psychological, and social aspects of individuals' lives. Recognizing this multifaceted nature, this guide endeavors to address not only the medical intricacies but also the holistic dimensions of living with and managing coronary heart disease.

In these pages, you'll find a wealth of information distilled from years of clinical experience, research endeavors, and patient interactions. From unraveling the intricate mechanisms underlying the disease to navigating the complexities of treatment modalities, each chapter endeavors to empower readers with knowledge, insight, and practical guidance.

While medical science continues to advance at a rapid pace, our understanding of coronary heart disease evolves incessantly. Thus, this guide is not a static repository of facts but rather a dynamic companion on your journey toward better health and well-being. It is my hope that the insights contained herein will serve as a beacon of knowledge, fostering informed decision-making, promoting proactive management, and ultimately enhancing the quality of life for those affected by coronary heart disease.

As you embark on this exploration, remember that you are not alone. Whether you are a patient seeking answers, a caregiver offering support, or a healthcare professional navigating the intricacies of treatment, know that a community of individuals stands united in the pursuit of better cardiovascular health.

Together, let us confront coronary heart disease with courage, resilience, and unwavering determination.

Warm regards,
Dr Elizabeth Williams

Chapter 1

Introduction to Coronary Heart Disease

Coronary heart disease (CHD) stands as one of the most prevalent and critical cardiovascular conditions worldwide, affecting millions of individuals each year. Understanding CHD begins with grasping its fundamental concepts, including its overview and the normal structure and function of the heart.

Overview

Coronary heart disease (CHD), also known as coronary artery disease (CAD), is a prevalent and potentially life-threatening condition characterized by the narrowing or blockage of the coronary arteries. These arteries supply oxygen-rich blood to the heart muscle, enabling it to function effectively.

The development of CHD is typically attributed to the accumulation of fatty deposits, cholesterol, and other substances within the coronary arteries, a process known as atherosclerosis. Over time, these deposits can restrict blood flow to the heart, leading to ischemia (a shortage of oxygen-rich blood) and subsequent damage to the heart muscle.

CHD often manifests as chest pain or discomfort, known as angina, although some individuals may experience no symptoms at all, a condition known as silent ischemia. In severe cases, CHD can precipitate myocardial infarction (heart attack) or even sudden cardiac death.

Several factors contribute to the development and progression of CHD, including high blood pressure, elevated cholesterol levels, diabetes, smoking, obesity, sedentary lifestyle, and family history of heart disease. Additionally, advancing age and genetic predisposition can increase an individual's susceptibility to CHD.

The diagnosis of CHD typically involves a combination of medical history assessment, physical examination, and diagnostic tests such as electrocardiography (ECG/EKG), stress testing, echocardiography, coronary angiography, and cardiac imaging studies.

Treatment strategies for CHD aim to alleviate symptoms, reduce the risk of complications, and improve overall cardiovascular health. These may include lifestyle modifications (such as dietary changes, regular exercise, smoking cessation, and stress management), medications (such as antiplatelet agents, beta-blockers, statins, and ACE inhibitors), and, in some cases, invasive procedures (such as angioplasty, stent placement, or coronary artery bypass grafting).

Prevention and management of CHD require a multifaceted approach, addressing modifiable risk factors, promoting healthy lifestyle choices, and fostering patient education and empowerment. By adopting proactive measures and adhering to recommended treatment regimens, individuals can mitigate the impact of CHD and enhance their quality of life.

Coronary heart disease remains a significant public health concern, exerting a considerable burden on individuals, healthcare systems, and society as a whole. Through concerted efforts in prevention, early detection, and comprehensive management, we can strive to mitigate the impact of CHD and improve cardiovascular outcomes for individuals worldwide.

Normal Structure and Function of the Heart

The heart is a muscle situated within the chest area, positioned slightly to the left of the centerline. It is responsible for pumping oxygen-rich blood throughout the body, ensuring the delivery of nutrients and removal of waste products.

Structurally, the heart comprises four chambers: two atria (upper chambers) and two ventricles (lower chambers). The right atrium receives deoxygenated blood from the body via the superior and inferior vena cavae and pumps it into the right ventricle. From there, the blood is pumped to the lungs for oxygenation. The left atrium receives oxygenated blood from the lungs via the pulmonary veins and pumps it into the left ventricle. The oxygenated blood is subsequently propelled to the rest of the body via the aorta by the left ventricle..

The heart is equipped with a specialized conduction system that coordinates its rhythmic contractions. The sinoatrial (SA) node, located in the right atrium, serves as the heart's natural pacemaker, generating electrical impulses that initiate each heartbeat. These signals move across the atria, prompting their contraction and pushing blood into the ventricles. The impulses then pass through the atrioventricular (AV) node, which delays their transmission to allow the ventricles to fill completely.

Subsequently, the impulses travel along the bundle of His and its branches, stimulating the ventricles to contract and eject blood into the pulmonary artery and aorta.

The cardiac cycle consists of two main phases: diastole and systole. During diastole, the heart relaxes, allowing the chambers to fill with blood. In systole, the heart contracts, expelling blood into the circulation. This rhythmic sequence of events ensures efficient blood flow and optimal cardiac output.

The heart is nourished by its own network of blood vessels, known as coronary arteries. These arteries originate from the aorta and encircle the heart, supplying it with oxygen and nutrients. Coronary artery disease, characterized by the narrowing or blockage of these arteries, can impair myocardial function and lead to complications such as angina, myocardial infarction, and heart failure.

The heart's intricate structure and coordinated function enable it to sustain life by maintaining circulation throughout the body. Understanding the normal anatomy and physiology of the heart lays the foundation for comprehending cardiovascular health and disease, guiding efforts to promote optimal cardiac function and well-being.

Chapter 2

Understanding Coronary Heart Disease

Coronary heart disease (CHD) is a complex cardiovascular condition that requires a thorough understanding of its causes, risk factors, types, and classification to effectively manage and prevent its progression.

Causes and Risk Factors

Coronary heart disease (CHD) arises from a complex interplay of genetic, environmental, and lifestyle factors. While the precise etiology may vary among individuals, several common causes and risk factors contribute to the development and progression of CHD:

- **Atherosclerosis**: The primary underlying cause of CHD is atherosclerosis, a condition characterized by the buildup of fatty deposits, cholesterol, and other substances within the walls of the coronary arteries. Over time, these deposits can narrow the arteries, restricting blood flow to the heart and increasing the risk of ischemia and myocardial infarction.

- **Hypertension (High Blood Pressure):** Elevated blood pressure exerts chronic strain on the arterial walls, promoting the development of atherosclerosis and increasing the risk of CHD. Hypertension also contributes to the progression of other cardiovascular conditions, such as heart failure and stroke.

- **Dyslipidemia (High Cholesterol):** Elevated levels of LDL cholesterol ("bad" cholesterol) and reduced levels of HDL cholesterol ("good" cholesterol) are associated with an increased risk of atherosclerosis and CHD. Excess LDL cholesterol can accumulate within the arterial walls, promoting plaque formation and arterial narrowing.

- **Diabetes Mellitus:** Individuals with diabetes are at heightened risk of developing CHD due to metabolic abnormalities that accelerate atherosclerosis and endothelial dysfunction. Poorly controlled blood sugar levels contribute to oxidative stress, inflammation, and vascular damage, further exacerbating cardiovascular risk.

- **Smoking:** Cigarette smoking is a major modifiable risk factor for CHD, exerting detrimental effects on cardiovascular health through multiple mechanisms. Smoking promotes endothelial dysfunction, vasoconstriction, platelet aggregation, and inflammation, all of which contribute to the development and progression of atherosclerosis.

- **Obesity and Sedentary Lifestyle**: Excess body weight, particularly abdominal adiposity, is associated with metabolic disturbances, insulin resistance, dyslipidemia, and hypertension, all of which increase the risk of CHD. Sedentary behavior exacerbates these risk factors, impairing cardiovascular fitness and promoting atherosclerosis.

- **Family History of CHD:** Genetic predisposition plays a significant role in the development of CHD, with individuals having a family history of premature heart disease being at higher risk. Inherited factors influence lipid metabolism, blood pressure regulation, thrombosis, and vascular function, contributing to familial clustering of CHD.

- **Age and Gender:** Advancing age is a non-modifiable risk factor for CHD, with the incidence and prevalence increasing with age. Men tend to develop CHD at a younger age than women, although the risk in postmenopausal women approaches that of men.

- **Other Risk Factors:** Additional risk factors for CHD include stress, poor dietary habits (high intake of saturated and trans fats, refined carbohydrates, and sodium), excessive alcohol consumption, sleep apnea, and certain medical conditions (e.g., chronic kidney disease, autoimmune disorders).

The development of CHD is influenced by a constellation of causes and risk factors, many of which are modifiable through lifestyle modifications, medication therapy, and targeted interventions. Identifying and addressing these risk factors early in life can mitigate the progression of atherosclerosis and reduce the burden of CHD, promoting cardiovascular health and longevity.

Types and Classification

Coronary heart disease (CHD) encompasses a spectrum of cardiovascular disorders characterized by the obstruction or narrowing of the coronary arteries, which supply oxygen-rich blood to the heart muscle. These conditions can be classified based on various criteria, including the underlying pathophysiology, clinical presentation, and severity of arterial involvement:

Atherosclerotic Coronary Artery Disease (CAD):

- Atherosclerosis, the gradual buildup of plaque within the coronary arteries, is the hallmark of CAD.

- CAD encompasses various manifestations, including stable angina, unstable angina, myocardial infarction (MI), and sudden cardiac death.

- **Stable angina** is characterized by predictable chest pain or discomfort triggered by exertion or emotional stress, usually relieved by rest or medication.

- **Unstable angina** refers to chest pain or discomfort that occurs at rest, with increasing frequency, duration, or severity, often indicating an acute coronary syndrome (ACS) and impending MI.

Acute Coronary Syndromes (ACS):
- ACS encompasses a spectrum of acute myocardial ischemic syndromes, ranging from unstable angina to non-ST-segment elevation MI (NSTEMI) and ST-segment elevation MI (STEMI).

- NSTEMI and STEMI represent distinct forms of MI, differentiated by the presence or absence of ST-segment elevation on electrocardiography.

- NSTEMI and unstable angina are often managed conservatively or with early invasive strategies, while STEMI requires emergent reperfusion therapy to restore blood flow to the ischemic myocardium.

Chronic Total Occlusion (CTO):
- CTO refers to the complete occlusion of a coronary artery, typically lasting for more than three months.

- CTOs may be asymptomatic or manifest as chronic stable angina, with symptoms often alleviated by collateral blood flow and medical therapy.

- Percutaneous coronary intervention (PCI) or coronary artery bypass grafting (CABG) may be considered for symptomatic patients with CTO, depending on the extent and severity of ischemia.

Microvascular Coronary Dysfunction (MCD):

- MCD is characterized by impaired coronary microvascular function, resulting in myocardial ischemia despite angiographically normal coronary arteries.

- MCD is more common in women and is associated with risk factors such as diabetes, hypertension, and systemic inflammation.

- Diagnosis of MCD often requires invasive coronary reactivity testing to assess microvascular function and guide therapeutic interventions.

Coronary Artery Spasm:

- Coronary artery spasm is characterized by transient episodes of intense vasoconstriction, leading to myocardial ischemia and angina.

- Spasms may occur spontaneously or be triggered by various factors, including emotional stress, exposure to cold temperatures, or certain medications.

- Calcium channel blockers and nitrates are the mainstays of treatment for coronary artery spasm, aimed at relieving symptoms and preventing recurrent episodes.

- CHD encompasses a diverse array of cardiovascular disorders, each with distinct pathophysiological mechanisms, clinical presentations, and management strategies. Understanding the types and classification of CHD is essential for accurate diagnosis, risk stratification, and personalized treatment planning, with the ultimate goal of improving patient outcomes and reducing the burden of cardiovascular morbidity and mortality.

Stages of Coronary Heart Disease

Coronary heart disease (CHD) progresses through various stages, each characterized by distinct pathophysiological changes, clinical manifestations, and prognostic implications. Understanding the stages of CHD is crucial for risk assessment, treatment planning, and monitoring of disease progression. The stages of CHD can be broadly categorized as follows:

Early Stage / Asymptomatic Phase:

- In the early stages of CHD, individuals may have underlying atherosclerosis without overt symptoms.

- Atherosclerosis progresses silently, with the gradual accumulation of plaque within the coronary arteries.

- Early detection of atherosclerosis may be possible through imaging modalities such as coronary artery calcium scoring or carotid intima-media thickness measurement.

- Lifestyle modifications, including dietary changes, regular exercise, smoking cessation, and optimal management of risk factors (e.g., hypertension, hyperlipidemia, diabetes), are critical for preventing disease progression and reducing cardiovascular risk.

Symptomatic Phase / Stable Angina:
- Stable angina is a common manifestation of CHD, characterized by predictable chest pain or discomfort precipitated by exertion or emotional stress.

- Symptoms typically resolve with rest or nitroglycerin administration and are reproducible with exertion.

- Stable angina reflects an imbalance between myocardial oxygen supply and demand, secondary to coronary artery stenosis or obstruction.

- Treatment strategies for stable angina focus on symptom relief, risk factor modification, and secondary prevention measures.

Acute Coronary Syndromes (ACS):

- ACS encompasses a spectrum of acute myocardial ischemic syndromes, including unstable angina, non-ST-segment elevation myocardial infarction (NSTEMI), and ST-segment elevation myocardial infarction (STEMI).

- Unstable angina is characterized by new-onset or worsening chest pain at rest, often indicative of plaque instability and impending myocardial infarction.

- NSTEMI and STEMI represent different forms of acute myocardial infarction, distinguished by the presence or absence of ST-segment elevation on electrocardiography.

- Prompt diagnosis and management of ACS are paramount, with timely reperfusion therapy (e.g., percutaneous coronary intervention, thrombolytic therapy) indicated for patients with STEMI.

Chronic Complications / Heart Failure and Arrhythmias:

- Chronic complications of CHD may include heart failure, arrhythmias, and sudden cardiac death.

- Chronic myocardial ischemia and infarction can lead to myocardial remodeling, impaired contractility, and progressive deterioration of cardiac function.

- Arrhythmias, including ventricular tachycardia, ventricular fibrillation, and atrial fibrillation, may occur secondary to myocardial ischemia, scar formation, or electrical remodeling.

- Management of chronic complications involves optimization of medical therapy, device-based therapies (e.g., implantable cardioverter-defibrillator, cardiac resynchronization therapy), and lifestyle modifications to improve symptoms and reduce morbidity and mortality.

The stages of coronary heart disease encompass a continuum of disease progression, from asymptomatic atherosclerosis to symptomatic angina, acute coronary syndromes, and chronic complications such as heart failure and arrhythmias. Early detection, risk factor modification, and timely intervention are essential for mitigating the impact of CHD and improving long-term outcomes for affected individuals.

Chapter 3

Signs and Symptoms

Common Symptoms of Coronary Heart Disease

Coronary heart disease (CHD) can manifest through various symptoms, which may vary in severity and presentation among individuals. Recognizing these symptoms is crucial for timely diagnosis, intervention, and management of CHD. Common symptoms of CHD include:

Angina Pectoris:
- Angina is the most characteristic symptom of CHD and often presents as chest discomfort or pressure.
- The sensation may also be described as squeezing, heaviness, tightness, or burning in the chest.

- Angina typically occurs during physical exertion, emotional stress, or exposure to cold temperatures and is relieved with rest or nitroglycerin.

Shortness of Breath (Dyspnea):
- Dyspnea, or difficulty breathing, may occur with exertion or at rest and is often indicative of underlying myocardial ischemia or heart failure.
- Individuals may experience a sensation of breathlessness, tightness in the chest, or inability to catch their breath.

Fatigue and weakness:
- Fatigue is a common symptom of CHD and may occur due to reduced cardiac output, myocardial ischemia, or underlying heart failure.
- Individuals may feel unusually tired, weak, or exhausted, even with minimal exertion or activity.

Palpitations:

- Palpitations refer to an abnormal awareness of the heartbeat, often described as rapid, irregular, or pounding.
- Palpitations may result from arrhythmias such as atrial fibrillation, ventricular tachycardia, or premature ventricular contractions, which can occur secondary to CHD.

Chest Discomfort:

- Chest discomfort associated with CHD may radiate to the arms, shoulders, neck, jaw, or back.
- The discomfort may be diffuse or localized and may worsen with exertion, emotional stress, or after heavy meals.

Nausea and Indigestion:

- Some individuals with CHD may experience symptoms of nausea, indigestion, or abdominal discomfort, which may mimic gastrointestinal disturbances.

- These symptoms may occur concurrently with chest pain or independently and may be attributed to reduced blood flow to the gastrointestinal organs.

Dizziness or Lightheadedness:
- Dizziness or lightheadedness may occur in individuals with CHD, particularly during episodes of reduced cardiac output or arrhythmias.
- These symptoms may be exacerbated by changes in posture, exertion, or dehydration.

Syncope (Fainting):
- Syncope, or fainting, may occur in severe cases of CHD, particularly during episodes of profound myocardial ischemia, arrhythmias, or hemodynamic instability.
- Syncope requires prompt evaluation to identify and address the underlying cause.

Sweating:

Sweating:

- Profuse sweating, particularly without exertion or in cool environments, may signal an underlying cardiac problem.

It is important to note that not all individuals with CHD will experience classic symptoms, and some may present with atypical or silent manifestations. Prompt evaluation by a healthcare professional is essential for accurate diagnosis and appropriate management of CHD and its associated symptoms.

Atypical Symptoms of Coronary Heart Disease

Coronary heart disease (CHD) can manifest through a spectrum of symptoms, including atypical presentations that may not immediately raise suspicion of cardiovascular involvement. Recognizing these atypical symptoms is crucial for identifying individuals at risk and facilitating early intervention and management. Common atypical symptoms of CHD include:

Silent Ischemia:

- Silent ischemia refers to a lack of symptoms despite reduced blood flow to the heart muscle.
- Individuals with silent ischemia may be asymptomatic or experience subtle symptoms that are easily overlooked.

Jaw Pain or Discomfort:

- Jaw pain or discomfort, particularly in the lower jaw, may occur in some individuals experiencing myocardial ischemia or angina.
- The sensation may be described as pressure, tightness, or aching and may radiate from the chest to the jaw.

Upper Back Pain:

- Upper back pain, between the shoulder blades or in the region of the shoulder blades, may be a manifestation of myocardial ischemia or angina.
- The pain may be intermittent or persistent and may worsen with exertion or emotional stress.

Shoulder Pain:

- Pain or discomfort in one or both shoulders, especially the left shoulder, may be associated with CHD.
- The pain may be dull, achy, or sharp and may occur at rest or during physical activity.

Arm Pain or Numbness:

- Pain, numbness, or tingling sensations in the arms, particularly the left arm, may occur in individuals experiencing myocardial ischemia or angina.
- The discomfort may extend from the chest to the arm, elbow, wrist, or fingers.

Neck Pain or Tightness:

- Neck pain or tightness, often described as a sensation of pressure or constriction, may occur in conjunction with chest discomfort in individuals with CHD.
- The discomfort may radiate from the chest to the neck or may be localized to the neck region.

Shortness of Breath (Dyspnea) without Chest Pain:

- Dyspnea, or difficulty breathing, may occur as an isolated symptom in individuals with CHD, particularly in the absence of chest pain.
- Dyspnea may be exertional or occur at rest and may be indicative of underlying myocardial ischemia, heart failure, or pulmonary congestion.

Unexplained Fatigue or Weakness:

- Unexplained fatigue or weakness, disproportionate to exertion or activity level, may be a subtle manifestation of CHD.
- Individuals may experience a sense of exhaustion, malaise, or diminished stamina without an obvious cause.

Epigastric Discomfort or Indigestion:

- Epigastric discomfort, indigestion, or heartburn-like symptoms may occur in some individuals with CHD, mimicking gastrointestinal disturbances.
- The discomfort may be mistaken for gastric reflux, gastritis, or peptic ulcer disease.

While atypical symptoms of CHD may not immediately raise suspicion of cardiovascular involvement, they should not be overlooked, particularly in individuals with known risk factors or predisposing conditions. Prompt evaluation by a healthcare professional is essential for accurate diagnosis and appropriate management of CHD and its associated symptoms.

Chapter 4

Diagnosis and Testing

Accurate diagnosis of coronary heart disease (CHD) relies on a combination of physical examination findings and diagnostic tests. Understanding the role of both components is essential in effectively evaluating patients for CHD and guiding appropriate management strategies.

Physical Examination

The physical examination plays a vital role in the evaluation of individuals suspected or diagnosed with coronary heart disease (CHD). While the diagnosis of CHD relies heavily on clinical history and diagnostic tests, certain physical findings can provide valuable insights into the cardiovascular status of the patient. Key components of the physical examination in CHD evaluation include:

- Measurement of vital signs, including blood pressure, heart rate, respiratory rate, and temperature, provides baseline information about the patient's hemodynamic status and overall cardiovascular health.
- Hypertension, tachycardia, and abnormal temperature may indicate underlying systemic inflammation or hemodynamic instability.

Cardiovascular Examination:

- Inspection, palpation, and auscultation of the heart provide important clues regarding cardiac structure, function, and rhythm.
- Inspection of the precordium may reveal visible pulsations, heaves, or lifts suggestive of cardiac hypertrophy or enlargement.
- Palpation of the chest may detect abnormal thrills, vibrations, or palpable impulses associated with cardiac pathology.

- Auscultation of the heart allows for assessment of heart sounds, murmurs, rubs, and gallops indicative of valvular abnormalities, myocardial dysfunction, or arrhythmias.

Peripheral Vascular Examination:
- Evaluation of peripheral pulses, capillary refill, and arterial and venous circulation provides information about peripheral perfusion and vascular integrity.
- Absent or diminished peripheral pulses, prolonged capillary refill, and signs of peripheral edema may suggest impaired arterial or venous circulation secondary to CHD or related comorbidities.

Respiratory Examination:
- Assessment of respiratory effort, lung auscultation, and percussion aids in identifying signs of pulmonary congestion, respiratory distress, or underlying lung pathology.

- Crackles, wheezes, or diminished breath sounds may indicate pulmonary congestion, pleural effusion, or chronic lung disease associated with CHD complications.

Peripheral Edema and Fluid Status:

- Inspection and palpation of the extremities for signs of peripheral edema, swelling, or fluid retention may indicate volume overload, heart failure, or venous insufficiency secondary to CHD.

Nutritional and Anthropometric Assessment:

- Evaluation of nutritional status, body mass index (BMI), waist circumference, and body composition provides insights into cardiovascular risk factors, metabolic health, and potential obesity-related complications.

Neurological Examination:

- Assessment of neurological status, including mental status, cranial nerves, motor function, and sensory perception, helps identify signs of cerebrovascular disease, cognitive impairment, or neurologic deficits associated with CHD complications.

The physical examination serves as a valuable adjunct to clinical history and diagnostic testing in the evaluation of CHD, providing clinicians with important diagnostic, prognostic, and therapeutic insights. Careful observation, systematic assessment, and attention to detail are essential for recognizing subtle signs and symptoms suggestive of underlying cardiovascular pathology and guiding optimal management strategies for patients with CHD.

Diagnostic Tests

Several diagnostic tests are available to evaluate individuals suspected of having coronary heart disease (CHD). These tests aim to assess cardiac structure, function, perfusion, and electrical activity, aiding in the diagnosis, risk stratification, and management of CHD. Key diagnostic tests include:

Electrocardiogram (ECG):

- An ECG records the electrical activity of the heart and helps identify abnormal rhythms, conduction disturbances, ischemic changes, and structural abnormalities.
- ST-segment elevation or depression, T-wave inversions, and pathological Q-waves may suggest myocardial ischemia, infarction, or prior myocardial injury.
- ECG findings may aid in diagnosing acute coronary syndromes, arrhythmias, myocardial hypertrophy, and conduction abnormalities associated with CHD.

Stress Test (Exercise Electrocardiogram):

- A stress test evaluates cardiovascular responses to physical exertion and helps detect ischemia, exercise-induced arrhythmias, and functional limitations.
- Exercise or pharmacological stress testing may be performed in individuals unable to exercise adequately.

- Ischemic changes on the ECG during stress (e.g., ST-segment depression) or symptoms such as chest pain or dyspnea may indicate underlying CHD.

Echocardiography (Echo):

- Echocardiography uses ultrasound waves to visualize cardiac structure, function, and blood flow dynamics.
- Echo assesses left ventricular size and function, valvular abnormalities, wall motion abnormalities, chamber dimensions, and intracardiac pressures.
- Echocardiography aids in the diagnosis of myocardial infarction, heart failure, valvular heart disease, and congenital heart defects associated with CHD.

Nuclear Cardiac Imaging (Myocardial Perfusion Imaging):

- Nuclear cardiac imaging involves the injection of radioactive tracers to assess myocardial perfusion and identify areas of ischemia or infarction.

- Stress and rest perfusion scans using single-photon emission computed tomography (SPECT) or positron emission tomography (PET) provide valuable information about myocardial viability and ischemic burden.

- Coronary angiography is the gold standard for diagnosing coronary artery disease and involves the injection of contrast dye into the coronary arteries followed by X-ray imaging.
- Angiography visualizes the location, severity, and extent of coronary artery stenosis, occlusion, or dissection.
- Coronary angiography helps guide treatment decisions, including percutaneous coronary intervention (PCI) with balloon angioplasty and stent placement or coronary artery bypass grafting (CABG) for revascularization.

Cardiac CT Angiography (CCTA):
- Cardiac CT angiography uses computed tomography (CT) imaging to visualize coronary artery anatomy, detect stenosis, and assess plaque burden.
- CCTA is a non-invasive alternative to conventional coronary angiography and provides detailed anatomical information about coronary arteries, bypass grafts, and cardiac structures.

Cardiac Magnetic Resonance Imaging (MRI):
- Cardiac MRI combines magnetic fields and radio waves to produce high-resolution images of the heart, blood vessels, and surrounding structures.
- MRI is valuable for assessing myocardial viability, myocardial perfusion, tissue characterization, and cardiac function.
- Cardiac MRI aids in the diagnosis and management of CHD, myocardial infarction, myocarditis, cardiomyopathies, and congenital heart defects.

- Blood tests, including lipid profile, cardiac biomarkers (troponin), and markers of inflammation (C-reactive protein), help assess cardiovascular risk, diagnose myocardial infarction, and monitor treatment response.

These diagnostic tests play a pivotal role in the comprehensive evaluation and management of individuals with suspected or established coronary heart disease.

By combining physical examination findings with appropriate diagnostic tests, healthcare providers can accurately diagnose CHD, assess its severity, and formulate individualized treatment plans tailored to each patient's specific needs and clinical presentation. Early diagnosis and intervention are key in optimizing outcomes and improving quality of life for individuals with CHD.

Chapter 5

Treatment Options

Addressing coronary heart disease (CHD) involves a multifaceted approach that includes medications and surgical procedures aimed at alleviating symptoms, improving cardiac function, and reducing the risk of cardiovascular events.

Medications

-Antiplatelet Agents

Antiplatelet agents play a crucial role in the management of coronary heart disease (CHD) by preventing platelet aggregation and thrombus formation, thereby reducing the risk of cardiovascular events such as myocardial infarction (MI) and stroke. Key antiplatelet agents used in CHD management include:

- Aspirin irreversibly inhibits cyclooxygenase (COX) enzymes, thereby blocking the synthesis of thromboxane A2, a potent platelet aggregator.
- Aspirin is considered the cornerstone of antiplatelet therapy in CHD and is recommended for secondary prevention in patients with a history of MI, unstable angina, percutaneous coronary intervention (PCI), or coronary artery bypass grafting (CABG).
- Low-dose aspirin (81 mg to 100 mg daily) is typically prescribed for long-term use in CHD patients, as higher doses are associated with an increased risk of gastrointestinal bleeding.

- P2Y12 inhibitors block the P2Y12 receptor on platelets, preventing adenosine diphosphate (ADP)-mediated platelet activation and aggregation.

- Clopidogrel, prasugrel, and ticagrelor are the main P2Y12 inhibitors used in CHD management.
- Clopidogrel is commonly prescribed in combination with aspirin for dual antiplatelet therapy (DAPT) following PCI with stent placement or in patients with acute coronary syndromes.
- Prasugrel and ticagrelor are more potent and rapid-acting P2Y12 inhibitors and may be preferred in high-risk patients with acute coronary syndromes undergoing PCI.

Glycoprotein IIb/IIIa Inhibitors:
- Glycoprotein IIb/IIIa inhibitors, such as abciximab, eptifibatide, and tirofiban, block the final common pathway of platelet aggregation by binding to the glycoprotein IIb/IIIa receptor on platelets.
- These agents are typically used as adjunctive therapy during PCI procedures to reduce the risk of periprocedural thrombotic complications, particularly in patients with high-risk features or complex coronary lesions.

Dual Antiplatelet Therapy (DAPT):

- DAPT refers to the concurrent use of aspirin and a P2Y12 inhibitor for a defined duration following PCI, acute coronary syndromes, or coronary artery stenting.
- DAPT reduces the risk of stent thrombosis, recurrent MI, and cardiovascular events compared to aspirin alone.
- The duration of DAPT varies depending on individual patient characteristics, stent type, and bleeding risk, with shorter durations favored in low-risk patients to minimize bleeding complications.

Adverse Effects and Monitoring:

- Antiplatelet agents are associated with an increased risk of bleeding, particularly gastrointestinal and intracranial bleeding.
- Patients receiving antiplatelet therapy should be monitored for signs of bleeding, including hematuria, melena, ecchymosis, and neurological deficits.
- Individualized assessment of bleeding and ischemic risks is essential to balance the benefits and risks of antiplatelet therapy in CHD patients.

Beta-blockers are medications used in various cardiovascular conditions, including coronary heart disease (CHD), hypertension, heart failure, and arrhythmias. They work by blocking the effects of adrenaline and other stress hormones on the heart and blood vessels. Key points about beta-blockers include:

Mechanism of Action:

- Beta-blockers block the beta-adrenergic receptors in the heart and blood vessels, reducing the effects of adrenaline and noradrenaline.
- By blocking these receptors, beta-blockers decrease heart rate, blood pressure, and myocardial contractility, reducing the workload on the heart.

Indications:

- In CHD, beta-blockers are used to reduce symptoms of angina (chest pain), improve exercise tolerance, and prevent heart attacks.

- They are also used after heart attacks to reduce the risk of future events and improve survival.
- Beta-blockers are beneficial in heart failure by reducing symptoms and improving heart function.

Types:
There are different types of beta-blockers, including selective (beta-1) blockers and non-selective blockers.

- Selective beta-1 blockers primarily affect the heart, while non-selective blockers also affect other organs like the lungs and blood vessels.

Examples include:
- Selective Beta-1 Blockers:
- Atenolol
- Metoprolol
- Bisoprolol
- Non-selective Beta-Blockers:
- Propranolol
- Carvedilol

- Beta-blockers reduce the heart's oxygen demand, making them effective in reducing angina symptoms and preventing heart attacks.
- They also help in controlling blood pressure and reducing the risk of arrhythmias.
- In heart failure, beta-blockers improve heart function and reduce the risk of hospitalization and death.

- Common side effects of beta-blockers include fatigue, dizziness, low blood pressure, and worsening of heart failure symptoms.
- They may also cause bronchospasm in patients with asthma or chronic obstructive pulmonary disease (COPD).
- Abrupt withdrawal of beta-blockers can lead to rebound hypertension and worsening of angina symptoms.

- Patients starting beta-blockers should be monitored for heart rate, blood pressure, and symptoms like dizziness or shortness of breath.

- Dosages may need adjustment based on individual response and tolerance.

Beta-blockers are valuable medications in the management of CHD and other cardiovascular conditions. They help reduce symptoms, prevent complications, and improve outcomes in patients with heart disease. However, careful monitoring and consideration of individual factors are important to ensure their safe and effective use.

–ACE Inhibitors

Angiotensin-converting enzyme (ACE) inhibitors are a class of medications used primarily in the management of cardiovascular conditions, including hypertension, heart failure, and coronary artery disease. Key points about ACE inhibitors include:

Mechanism of Action:

- ACE inhibitors block the activity of angiotensin-converting enzymes, which convert angiotensin I to angiotensin II.
- By inhibiting angiotensin II production, ACE inhibitors reduce vasoconstriction, aldosterone secretion, sodium and water retention, and sympathetic activation.
- These actions result in vasodilation, decreased blood pressure, and reduced cardiac workload, making ACE inhibitors effective in managing hypertension and heart failure.

Indications:

- ACE inhibitors are first-line agents for the treatment of hypertension and are recommended in patients with heart failure with reduced ejection fraction (HFrEF) to improve symptoms and reduce mortality.
- They are also indicated in patients with left ventricular dysfunction following myocardial infarction to prevent adverse cardiac remodeling and reduce the risk of heart failure and mortality.

Commonly prescribed ACE inhibitors include:

- Enalapril
- Lisinopril
- Ramipril
- Captopril
- Benazepril
- Perindopril
- Fosinopril

- ACE inhibitors effectively lower blood pressure by dilating blood vessels, reducing afterload, and improving systemic vascular resistance.
- In heart failure, ACE inhibitors improve symptoms, reduce hospitalizations, and prolong survival by attenuating neurohormonal activation and ventricular remodeling.
- They have renoprotective effects and are beneficial in patients with diabetic nephropathy or chronic kidney disease.

- Common side effects of ACE inhibitors include dry cough, hyperkalemia, hypotension, dizziness, and renal dysfunction.
- ACE inhibitors should be used cautiously in patients with bilateral renal artery stenosis, hyperkalemia, or a history of angioedema, as they may exacerbate these conditions.
- Pregnancy is a contraindication for ACE inhibitor use due to the risk of fetal harm, including renal dysfunction and fetal death.

Monitoring:

- Patients starting ACE inhibitors should undergo regular monitoring of renal function, potassium levels, and blood pressure.
- Dosages may need adjustment based on individual response and tolerability.

ACE inhibitors are cornerstone medications in the management of hypertension, heart failure, and other cardiovascular conditions. They offer significant benefits in reducing blood pressure, improving cardiac function, and preventing adverse outcomes in high-risk patients. Careful selection, dosing, and monitoring of ACE inhibitor therapy are essential to optimize clinical outcomes and minimize adverse effects.

–Statins

Statins are a class of medications primarily used to lower cholesterol levels and reduce the risk of cardiovascular events. Key points about statins include:

Mechanism of Action:
- Statins inhibit the enzyme HMG-CoA reductase, which is involved in cholesterol synthesis in the liver.
- By inhibiting cholesterol production, statins increase the number of LDL receptors on liver cells, leading to enhanced removal of LDL cholesterol from the bloodstream.
- Statins also have anti-inflammatory and plaque-stabilizing effects, contributing to their cardiovascular benefits beyond cholesterol lowering.

- Statins are indicated for the primary and secondary prevention of cardiovascular events, including heart attacks, strokes, and coronary artery disease.
- They are prescribed to individuals with high cholesterol levels, especially those with a history of cardiovascular disease, diabetes, or other risk factors.

Examples:
Commonly prescribed statins include:

- Atorvastatin
- Simvastatin
- Rosuvastatin
- Pravastatin
- Fluvastatin
- Lovastatin
- Pitavastatin

Benefits:

- Statins effectively lower LDL cholesterol levels, which are a major risk factor for atherosclerosis and cardiovascular disease.

- They also modestly increase HDL cholesterol levels and reduce triglycerides.
- Statins have been shown to reduce the risk of heart attacks, strokes, and cardiovascular mortality in both primary and secondary prevention settings.
- They are associated with improvements in endothelial function, plaque stabilization, and reduction in inflammation within the arterial wall.

Adverse Effects:
- Common side effects of statins include muscle pain, weakness, and elevated liver enzymes.
- Severe side effects such as rhabdomyolysis (muscle breakdown) and liver damage are rare but can occur, especially at higher doses.
- Statins may also slightly increase the risk of developing diabetes mellitus, although the cardiovascular benefits generally outweigh this risk.

Monitoring:

- Patients starting statin therapy should undergo baseline liver function tests and periodic monitoring of liver enzymes.
- Muscle symptoms should be promptly reported to healthcare providers for evaluation, and statin therapy may need to be adjusted or discontinued if symptoms persist.

Statins are highly effective medications for lowering cholesterol levels and reducing the risk of cardiovascular events. They are widely used in clinical practice and have been shown to improve outcomes in patients with or at risk of cardiovascular disease. However, careful monitoring and management of side effects are important aspects of statin therapy to ensure optimal safety and efficacy.

–Others

In addition to Antiplatelet Agents, Statins, Beta-blockers, and ACE inhibitors, several other medications play important roles in the management of coronary heart disease (CHD). Key points about these medications include:

Calcium Channel Blockers:
- Calcium channel blockers, including diltiazem and verapamil, are used to reduce blood pressure and control angina symptoms in patients with CHD.
- They dilate coronary arteries, improve myocardial oxygen supply, and reduce myocardial oxygen demand, making them effective in angina management.

Nitrates:
- Nitrates, such as nitroglycerin, provide rapid relief of angina symptoms by dilating coronary arteries and improving myocardial blood flow.
- They are available in various formulations, including sublingual tablets, sprays, and patches, for immediate or sustained symptom relief.

Diuretics:

- Diuretics, such as furosemide and hydrochlorothiazide, are used to reduce fluid retention and lower blood pressure in patients with heart failure and volume overload.
- They promote diuresis and sodium excretion, reducing cardiac preload and alleviating symptoms of congestion and edema.

Stable Nitric Oxide Donors:

- Stable nitric oxide donors, such as isosorbide dinitrate and isosorbide mononitrate, are used for the prevention and treatment of angina pectoris.
- They release nitric oxide, a potent vasodilator, which relaxes vascular smooth muscle and improves coronary blood flow.

Angiotensin II Receptor Blockers (ARBs):

- ARBs, including losartan and valsartan, block the effects of angiotensin II by selectively antagonizing angiotensin II type 1 receptors.

- They are used in patients intolerant to ACE inhibitors or as alternatives in the management of hypertension and heart failure.

Potassium-Sparing Diuretics:

- Potassium-sparing diuretics, such as spironolactone and eplerenone, inhibit aldosterone receptors and promote sodium excretion while conserving potassium.
- They are used as adjunctive therapy in patients with heart failure and as potassium-sparing alternatives to traditional diuretics.

These medications, along with lifestyle modifications and other interventions, constitute a comprehensive approach to managing coronary heart disease. Treatment strategies are tailored to individual patient characteristics, including disease severity, comorbidities, and medication tolerance, with the goal of reducing symptoms, preventing complications, and improving overall quality of life.

Surgical Procedures in Coronary Heart Disease Management

Surgical interventions play a crucial role in the management of coronary heart disease (CHD), particularly in patients with significant coronary artery blockages or complex coronary anatomy. Key surgical procedures include angioplasty and stent placement, as well as coronary artery bypass grafting (CABG). Here's an overview:

Angioplasty and Stent Placement:
- Angioplasty, also known as percutaneous coronary intervention (PCI), is a minimally invasive procedure used to open narrowed or blocked coronary arteries.
- During angioplasty, a catheter with a balloon at its tip is inserted into the narrowed artery and inflated to compress the plaque and widen the vessel lumen.
- Stent placement is often performed concurrently with angioplasty to help maintain the patency of the treated artery.

- Stents are small mesh tubes inserted into the artery to provide structural support and prevent restenosis (re-narrowing) of the vessel.
- Drug-eluting stents, coated with medications to inhibit cell proliferation, are commonly used to further reduce the risk of restenosis.

Angioplasty and stent placement are effective in relieving symptoms of angina, improving exercise tolerance, and reducing the risk of myocardial infarction in selected patients with CHD.

Coronary Artery Bypass Grafting (CABG):
- CABG is a surgical procedure used to bypass obstructed coronary arteries and restore blood flow to the heart muscle.
- During CABG, a healthy artery or vein from another part of the body, typically the chest wall or leg, is harvested and grafted onto the coronary artery beyond the blockage.

- The grafted vessel bypasses the blocked segment of the coronary artery, allowing blood to flow freely to the heart muscle.
- CABG is indicated in patients with severe multivessel coronary artery disease, left main coronary artery disease, or failed PCI with diffuse disease.
- It is also performed in patients with unstable angina or acute myocardial infarction who are not suitable candidates for PCI.

CABG is associated with excellent long-term outcomes, including symptom relief, improved quality of life, and reduced mortality in selected patients with CHD.

Implantable Cardioverter-Defibrillator (ICD):

- ICDs are implanted devices that deliver electrical shocks or pacing to restore normal heart rhythm and prevent sudden cardiac death in patients at high risk of life-threatening arrhythmias.

- **Cardiac Rehabilitation:**
  Cardiac rehabilitation programs offer comprehensive multidisciplinary interventions, including exercise training, education, counseling, and psychosocial support, to optimize recovery and improve outcomes in individuals with CHD.

These surgical procedures, angioplasty and stent placement, and coronary artery bypass grafting, are integral components of the treatment armamentarium for coronary heart disease. The selection of the appropriate intervention depends on individual patient characteristics, including disease severity, anatomy, comorbidities, and procedural risks. Timely and judicious use of surgical interventions can alleviate symptoms, improve cardiac function, and enhance overall prognosis in patients with CHD.

By combining pharmacological therapy with appropriate surgical interventions and lifestyle modifications, healthcare providers can effectively manage CHD, alleviate symptoms, and improve quality of life for patients living with this condition. Tailoring treatment plans to individual patient needs and preferences ensures optimal outcomes and patient satisfaction.

Complications of Coronary Heart Disease

Coronary heart disease (CHD) can lead to various complications that may significantly impact an individual's health and quality of life. Understanding these complications is crucial for patients and healthcare providers in managing CHD and preventing adverse outcomes.

Myocardial Infarction (Heart Attack):

- Myocardial infarction occurs when a coronary artery becomes suddenly blocked, depriving a portion of the heart muscle of oxygen-rich blood.

- Complications of myocardial infarction include heart failure, arrhythmias, cardiogenic shock, and sudden cardiac death.

Heart Failure:
- Heart failure occurs when the heart is unable to pump blood effectively to meet the body's demands, leading to symptoms such as shortness of breath, fatigue, and fluid retention.
- CHD-related heart failure may result from myocardial infarction, ischemic cardiomyopathy, or chronic ischemia compromising cardiac function.

Arrhythmias:
- CHD can disrupt the heart's electrical system, leading to abnormal heart rhythms known as arrhythmias.
- Ventricular arrhythmias such as ventricular tachycardia and ventricular fibrillation can be life-threatening and may result in sudden cardiac arrest.

Stroke:

- Individuals with CHD are at increased risk of stroke, particularly if atherosclerosis affects the carotid arteries supplying blood to the brain.
- Stroke may occur as a result of embolus originating from plaque rupture in the carotid arteries or from atrial fibrillation associated with CHD.

Peripheral Artery Disease (PAD):

- PAD is a manifestation of atherosclerosis affecting the arteries supplying blood to the extremities, leading to reduced blood flow, intermittent claudication, and tissue ischemia.
- Individuals with CHD are at higher risk of PAD and its associated complications, including leg ulcers, gangrene, and limb amputation.

Sudden Cardiac Death:

- Sudden cardiac death refers to unexpected death due to cardiac causes, often occurring within an hour of symptom onset.

- CHD-related sudden cardiac death may result from lethal arrhythmias such as ventricular fibrillation, triggered by myocardial ischemia or scar tissue from previous myocardial infarction.

Bleeding Events:

- Antithrombotic medications such as antiplatelet agents and anticoagulants, used to prevent thrombotic events, can increase the risk of bleeding.
- Bleeding events may range from minor bruising to life-threatening hemorrhages, particularly in patients undergoing invasive procedures like angioplasty or coronary artery bypass grafting (CABG).

Psychological and Emotional Impact:

- Living with CHD can have profound psychological and emotional effects, including anxiety, depression, and decreased quality of life.

- Coping with the diagnosis, managing symptoms, and adjusting to lifestyle changes can be challenging for individuals with CHD and their families.

Understanding and addressing these complications require a comprehensive approach to CHD management, including risk factor modification, medical therapy, lifestyle interventions, and regular monitoring. Timely recognition and intervention can help mitigate the impact of complications and improve outcomes for individuals living with coronary heart disease.

Chapter 6

Management and Side Effects

Coronary heart disease (CHD) management involves addressing symptoms, managing side effects of medications and procedures, and mitigating complications associated with the condition.

Managing Symptoms of Coronary Heart Disease

Managing symptoms of coronary heart disease (CHD) is essential for improving quality of life and reducing the risk of cardiovascular events. Effective symptom management involves a combination of lifestyle modifications, medication therapy, and patient education tailored to each individual's needs.

- **Heart-Healthy Diet**: Adopting a diet rich in fruits, vegetables, whole grains, lean proteins, and healthy fats can help control cholesterol levels, blood pressure, and weight, reducing the strain on the heart and alleviating symptoms of CHD.
- **Regular Exercise:** Engaging in regular physical activity, as recommended by healthcare providers, improves cardiovascular fitness, reduces stress, and enhances overall well-being. Exercise also helps manage weight, blood pressure, and cholesterol levels.
- **Smoking Cessation**: Quitting smoking is crucial for individuals with CHD, as tobacco smoke damages blood vessels, increases the risk of blood clots, and worsens symptoms of angina and shortness of breath.
- **Stress Management:** Practicing stress-reduction techniques such as deep breathing exercises, meditation, yoga, and mindfulness can help alleviate

anxiety, reduce emotional distress, and improve coping mechanisms.

Medication Therapy:

- **Antiplatelet Agents:** Medications such as aspirin, clopidogrel, and ticagrelor inhibit platelet aggregation, reducing the risk of blood clot formation and preventing thrombotic events in individuals with CHD.
- **Beta-Blockers**: Beta-blockers such as metoprolol, carvedilol, and bisoprolol reduce heart rate, blood pressure, and myocardial oxygen demand, relieving symptoms of angina and improving exercise tolerance.
- **Nitroglycerin**: Nitroglycerin is a vasodilator medication that helps dilate coronary arteries, improving blood flow to the heart and relieving chest pain associated with angina.
- **Statins**: Statins such as atorvastatin, simvastatin, and rosuvastatin lower LDL cholesterol levels, stabilize atherosclerotic plaques, and reduce the

risk of cardiovascular events in patients with CHD.

- Providing comprehensive patient education about CHD, its symptoms, treatment options, and self-care strategies empowers individuals to actively participate in their care and make informed decisions.
- Encouraging open communication, regular follow-up visits, and adherence to treatment plans fosters trust, engagement, and collaboration between patients and healthcare providers.

By implementing lifestyle modifications, adhering to medication regimens, and staying informed about CHD management strategies, individuals can effectively manage symptoms, improve quality of life, and reduce the risk of complications associated with coronary heart disease. Ongoing support from healthcare providers, family members, and support groups further enhances the success of symptom management efforts.

Side Effects of Medications and Procedures:

While medications and procedures are essential components of coronary heart disease (CHD) management, they may be associated with potential side effects that individuals need to be aware of. Understanding these side effects allows patients and healthcare providers to weigh the benefits against the risks and make informed treatment decisions.

Side Effects of Medications:

Antiplatelet Agents:

- **Bleeding**: Antiplatelet medications such as aspirin and clopidogrel increase the risk of bleeding, particularly gastrointestinal bleeding and bruising.

- **Gastrointestinal Upset**: Some individuals may experience nausea, indigestion, or abdominal discomfort while taking antiplatelet agents.

Beta-Blockers:
- **Fatigue**: Beta-blockers can cause fatigue, lethargy, and drowsiness, which may impact daily activities and quality of life.
- **Bradycardia**: These medications may slow heart rate, leading to bradycardia (abnormally slow heart rhythm) in some individuals.

Nitroglycerin:
- **Headaches**: Nitroglycerin may cause headaches, particularly upon initiation of therapy or with higher doses.
- **Hypotension**: Rapid lowering of blood pressure (hypotension) may occur, especially when changing positions or with sudden exertion.

- **Muscle Pain**: Statins may cause muscle pain, weakness, or tenderness, known as statin-induced myopathy.
- **Liver Function Abnormalities**: Rarely, statins can cause liver enzyme abnormalities or liver damage, necessitating monitoring of liver function tests.

Renal Dysfunction:

- Certain medications, particularly ACE inhibitors and nonsteroidal anti-inflammatory drugs (NSAIDs), can impair renal function and exacerbate pre-existing kidney disease.
- Renal function should be monitored regularly in patients receiving these medications to detect and manage renal dysfunction promptly.

Electrolyte Imbalances:

- Diuretics, particularly loop diuretics, used in heart failure management can lead to electrolyte imbalances, including hypokalemia, hyponatremia, and hypomagnesemia.

- Electrolyte levels should be monitored regularly, and supplementation may be necessary to maintain electrolyte balance.

Hypotension:

- Medications such as ACE inhibitors, beta-blockers, and diuretics can lower blood pressure, leading to symptomatic hypotension, dizziness, and lightheadedness.
- Blood pressure should be monitored regularly, and medication dosages may need to be adjusted to prevent excessive hypotension.

Thrombotic Events:

- Despite antithrombotic therapy, patients with CHD remain at risk of thrombotic events, including myocardial infarction, stroke, and venous thromboembolism.

- Optimizing antithrombotic regimens and addressing modifiable risk factors are essential to reduce the risk of thrombotic complications.

Percutaneous Coronary Intervention (PCI):
- **Bleeding**: PCI carries a risk of bleeding, particularly at the site of catheter insertion in the groin or wrist.
- **Restenosis**: In-stent restenosis, the re-narrowing of the treated coronary artery, may occur months or years after PCI.

Coronary Artery Bypass Grafting (CABG):
- **Infection**: CABG is associated with a risk of surgical site infection, which may require antibiotic treatment or surgical intervention.
- **Bleeding and Blood Transfusion**: CABG surgery may result in significant blood loss, necessitating blood transfusion and

increasing the risk of postoperative complications.

Implantable Cardioverter-Defibrillator (ICD):

- **Device Complications**: ICD implantation carries a risk of device-related complications, including infection, lead dislodgement, and device malfunction.
- **Psychological Impact**: Living with an ICD may lead to psychological distress, anxiety, and depression in some individuals.

It is essential for patients to communicate any side effects or concerns with their healthcare providers promptly. Healthcare providers can then adjust medications, monitor for complications, and provide supportive care to minimize adverse effects and optimize treatment outcomes. Regular follow-up appointments and open dialogue between patients and healthcare providers are critical in managing side effects and ensuring the safe and effective use of medications and procedures for CHD management.

Also healthcare providers should discuss the risks and benefits of interventions with patients and obtain informed consent before proceeding with procedures.

Chapter 7

Nutrition and Diet for Coronary Heart Disease Management

Proper nutrition and dietary habits play a crucial role in the management and prevention of coronary heart disease (CHD). Understanding the importance of diet and making recommended dietary changes can significantly impact cardiovascular health.

Importance of Diet in Management

- Diet influences risk factors such as cholesterol levels, blood pressure, inflammation, and body weight, all of which are critical in CHD management.

- A heart-healthy diet can reduce the progression of atherosclerosis, stabilize plaque, and improve overall cardiovascular health.

- Dietary modifications complement medical therapy, enhancing treatment efficacy and reducing the risk of cardiovascular events.

Recommended Dietary Changes

Foods to Eat:
- **Fruits and Vegetables**: Rich in vitamins, minerals, antioxidants, and fiber, these foods reduce inflammation and lower cholesterol levels.

- **Whole Grains:** Brown rice, quinoa, oats, and whole wheat bread are high in fiber and stabilize blood sugar, improving cholesterol levels.

- **Healthy Fats**: Nuts, seeds, avocados, and fatty fish like salmon are rich in omega-3 fatty acids, which lower triglyceride levels and inflammation.

- **Lean Proteins:** Poultry without skin, fish, legumes, tofu, and low-fat dairy products are preferable over red and processed meats due to their lower saturated fat content.

- **Plant-Based Proteins:** Beans, lentils, chickpeas, and soy products are low in saturated fat and cholesterol, reducing the risk of heart disease.

Foods to Avoid:

- **Saturated and Trans Fats:** Limit fatty meats, full-fat dairy products, fried foods, and commercially baked goods to reduce LDL cholesterol levels.

- **Added Sugars and Refined Carbohydrates:** Minimize sugary drinks, desserts, candies, and refined carbohydrates to stabilize blood sugar levels and reduce insulin resistance.

- **High-Sodium Foods**: Avoid processed and packaged foods high in sodium, such as canned soups, processed meats, salty snacks, and fast food, to lower blood pressure.

Incorporating these dietary changes supports cardiovascular health, reduces the risk of CHD complications, and improves overall well-being. A heart-healthy diet is a cornerstone of CHD management and prevention, complementing lifestyle modifications and medical therapy.

Chapter 8

Exercise Guidelines for Coronary Heart Disease Management

Regular exercise is a cornerstone of coronary heart disease (CHD) management, offering numerous benefits for cardiovascular health. Understanding the benefits, types of exercises recommended, and precautions are essential for individuals with CHD.

Benefits of Exercise

- **Improved Cardiovascular Health:** Exercise strengthens the heart muscle, improves circulation, and enhances cardiac function, reducing the risk of heart attacks and strokes.

- **Lower Blood Pressure:** Regular physical activity helps lower blood pressure and improves blood vessel function, reducing strain on the heart and arteries.

- **Better Cholesterol Levels:** Exercise raises HDL (good) cholesterol levels and lowers LDL (bad) cholesterol levels, improving lipid profiles and reducing the risk of atherosclerosis.

- **Weight Management:** Physical activity helps control body weight and body fat, reducing the risk of obesity and metabolic syndrome.

- **Improved Mood and Mental Health**: Exercise releases endorphins, which promote feelings of well-being and reduce stress, anxiety, and depression.

- **Enhanced Quality of Life:** Regular exercise improves stamina, energy levels, and overall quality of life for individuals with CHD.

Types of Exercise Recommended

- **Aerobic Exercise:** Activities such as brisk walking, jogging, cycling, swimming, and dancing elevate heart rate and increase oxygen consumption, improving cardiovascular fitness.

- **Strength Training:** Resistance exercises using weights, resistance bands, or bodyweight exercises help build muscle strength and endurance, supporting overall physical function and stability.

- **Flexibility and Balance Exercises:** Stretching exercises, yoga, and tai chi enhance flexibility, joint mobility, and balance, reducing the risk of falls and injuries.

Precautions and Guidelines

- **Consultation with Healthcare Provider:** Individuals with CHD should consult their healthcare provider before starting an exercise program, especially if they have existing cardiovascular conditions or other health concerns.

- **Start Slowly and Progress Gradually:** Begin with low-intensity activities and gradually increase duration, frequency, and intensity over time to avoid overexertion and injury.

- **Listen to Your Body**: Pay attention to signs and symptoms such as chest pain, shortness of breath, dizziness, nausea, or palpitations during exercise. Stop activity and seek medical attention if any symptoms occur.

- **Stay Hydrated:** Drink plenty of water before, during, and after exercise to stay hydrated and prevent dehydration.

- **Warm-Up and Cool Down:** Always start with a warm-up session to prepare muscles and joints for exercise and end with a cool-down to gradually lower heart rate and prevent post-exercise hypotension.

- **Safety Precautions**: Wear appropriate footwear and clothing, choose safe and well-lit exercise environments, and use proper equipment to minimize the risk of injury.

Incorporating regular exercise into daily routines is essential for managing CHD, improving cardiovascular health, and enhancing overall well-being. Following these exercise guidelines, individuals can reap the benefits of physical activity while minimizing risks and optimizing safety.

Chapter 9

Prevention and Risk Reduction

Preventing coronary heart disease (CHD) and reducing risk factors are essential for maintaining cardiovascular health. Lifestyle modifications and effective management of risk factors play a crucial role in prevention strategies.

Lifestyle Changes in Coronary Heart Disease Management

Lifestyle modifications play a critical role in the management and prevention of coronary heart disease (CHD). Key lifestyle changes include:

Healthy Diet:
- Adopting a heart-healthy diet rich in fruits, vegetables, whole grains, lean proteins, and healthy fats can help

reduce cholesterol levels, blood pressure, and body weight.
- Limiting saturated fats, trans fats, cholesterol, sodium, and added sugars can lower the risk of atherosclerosis and cardiovascular events.

Regular Exercise:
- Engaging in regular physical activity, such as brisk walking, cycling, swimming, or aerobic exercise, improves cardiovascular fitness, strengthens the heart muscle, and helps control weight.
- Aim to engage in a minimum of 150 minutes of moderate-intensity aerobic exercise weekly, or 75 minutes of vigorous-intensity aerobic exercise, complemented by muscle-strengthening exercises on at least two days per week.

Smoking Cessation:
- Quitting smoking is one of the most important steps individuals can take to reduce the risk of CHD and improve overall health.

- Smoking cessation significantly lowers the risk of heart attacks, strokes, and peripheral artery disease and leads to immediate and long-term health benefits.

Weight Management:
- Maintaining a healthy weight through a balanced diet and regular physical activity helps reduce the risk factors associated with CHD, including hypertension, dyslipidemia, and diabetes.
- Achieving and maintaining a body mass index (BMI) within the normal range (18.5 to 24.9 kg/m²) is associated with improved cardiovascular outcomes.

Stress Management:
- Chronic stress can contribute to the development and progression of CHD by promoting inflammation, endothelial dysfunction, and adverse health behaviors.
- Stress-reduction techniques such as mindfulness meditation, deep breathing exercises, yoga, and relaxation therapies

can help alleviate stress and promote emotional well-being.

Limit Alcohol Intake:

- Excessive alcohol consumption can increase blood pressure, triglyceride levels, and the risk of arrhythmias and cardiomyopathy.
- Moderation is key, with recommended limits of up to one drink per day for women and up to two drinks per day for men.

Regular Medical Check-Ups:

- Regular visits to healthcare providers for preventive screenings, blood pressure monitoring, cholesterol checks, and diabetes management are essential for early detection and management of risk factors for CHD.

By incorporating these lifestyle changes into daily routines, individuals can reduce the risk of developing CHD, slow the progression of existing disease, and improve overall cardiovascular health. A comprehensive approach that combines medical therapy with lifestyle modifications is essential for optimal CHD management and prevention of cardiovascular events.

Risk Factor Management

- **Blood Pressure Control:** Monitor blood pressure regularly and take steps to lower high blood pressure through lifestyle modifications and medication adherence.

- **Lipid Management**: Monitor lipid levels, including LDL cholesterol, HDL cholesterol, and triglycerides, and manage dyslipidemia through diet, exercise, and medication therapy (e.g., statins).

- **Diabetes Management**: Control blood glucose levels through diet, exercise, medication adherence, and regular monitoring of blood sugar levels.

Optimize glycemic control to reduce the risk of cardiovascular complications.

- **Hypertension Management:** Control hypertension through lifestyle modifications and antihypertensive medications to reduce the risk of CHD, stroke, and other cardiovascular events.

- **Cholesterol Management:** Lower LDL cholesterol levels and raise HDL cholesterol levels through diet, exercise, and medication therapy as needed to reduce the risk of atherosclerosis and CHD.

By implementing these prevention strategies and effectively managing risk factors, individuals can reduce the likelihood of developing CHD and improve overall cardiovascular health. Regular medical check-ups, preventive screenings, and adherence to treatment guidelines are essential components of comprehensive CHD prevention and risk reduction efforts.

Chapter 10

Prognosis and Survival Rates

Understanding the prognosis and survival rates associated with coronary heart disease (CHD) is essential for patients and healthcare providers. Several factors influence prognosis, and survival rates provide valuable insights into the outcomes of CHD.

Factors Affecting Prognosis:

- **Disease Severity:** The extent and severity of coronary artery disease, including the presence of significant stenosis, plaque burden, and involvement of multiple vessels, impact prognosis.

- **Left Ventricular Function:** Impaired left ventricular function, as assessed by echocardiography or cardiac imaging techniques, is associated with poorer prognosis and increased risk of heart failure and cardiovascular events.

- **Comorbidities**: The presence of comorbid conditions such as diabetes mellitus, hypertension, chronic kidney disease, and peripheral artery disease complicates CHD management and influences prognosis.

- **Age and Gender:** Advanced age and male gender are associated with higher cardiovascular risk and worse prognosis in patients with CHD.

- **Risk Factor Control:** Effective management of modifiable risk factors such as hypertension, dyslipidemia, diabetes, obesity, smoking, and sedentary lifestyle improves prognosis and reduces the risk of adverse cardiovascular events.

- **Treatment Adherence:** Adherence to medical therapy, lifestyle modifications, and recommended interventions, including medication regimens, cardiac rehabilitation, and follow-up appointments, affects long-term outcomes and prognosis.

Survival Rates and Statistics:

- **Overall Survival Rates:** Survival rates for CHD have improved significantly over the years due to advances in medical therapy, interventional procedures, and lifestyle modifications.

- **Five-Year Survival Rates**: The five-year survival rate for individuals diagnosed with CHD varies depending on disease severity, comorbidities, and treatment strategies. Generally, the survival rate is favorable with timely diagnosis and appropriate management.

- **Long-Term Prognosis**: Long-term prognosis in CHD is influenced by factors such as disease progression, treatment response, development of complications, and adherence to recommended lifestyle and medical interventions.

- **Risk Stratification Models:** Risk stratification models, such as the Framingham Risk Score, the ASCVD Risk Calculator, and the GRACE Score, help assess individual cardiovascular risk and predict outcomes in patients with CHD.

Understanding the factors affecting prognosis and survival rates in CHD enables healthcare providers to tailor treatment strategies, monitor patients closely, and optimize long-term outcomes. Early detection, aggressive risk factor modification, and multidisciplinary care are crucial in improving prognosis and enhancing quality of life for individuals with CHD.

Chapter 11

Living with Coronary Heart Disease

Living with coronary heart disease (CHD) requires adopting coping strategies and accessing support resources to manage the condition effectively.

Coping Strategies

Education and Awareness: Understanding the nature of CHD, its risk factors, symptoms, treatment options, and prognosis empowers individuals to make informed decisions and actively participate in their care.

Adherence to Treatment Plans: Strict adherence to medication regimens, lifestyle modifications, and follow-up appointments is essential for managing CHD and preventing complications.

Stress Management: Practicing stress-reduction techniques such as deep breathing exercises, meditation, yoga, and mindfulness can help alleviate anxiety, reduce emotional distress, and promote emotional well-being.

Healthy Lifestyle Habits: Adopting a heart-healthy diet, engaging in regular physical activity, maintaining a healthy weight, avoiding tobacco use, and limiting alcohol consumption are fundamental to managing CHD and optimizing cardiovascular health.

Seeking Social Support: Building a strong support network of family, friends, healthcare providers, and support groups provides emotional support, encouragement, and practical assistance in coping with the challenges of CHD.

Positive Attitude and Resilience: Maintaining a positive attitude, practicing resilience, and focusing on achievable goals contribute to a sense of control, optimism, and empowerment in managing CHD.

Support Resources

-**Healthcare Providers:** Cardiologists, primary care physicians, nurses, dietitians, and other healthcare professionals play integral roles in providing medical care, education, guidance, and support to individuals living with CHD.

-**Cardiac Rehabilitation Programs:** Cardiac rehabilitation programs offer structured exercise programs, education sessions, lifestyle counseling, and emotional support to individuals recovering from CHD events or managing chronic cardiovascular conditions.

-**Support Groups:** Joining CHD support groups or online communities provides opportunities for individuals to connect with others facing similar challenges, share experiences, exchange information, and offer mutual support and encouragement.

-Patient Advocacy Organizations: National and local patient advocacy organizations, such as the American Heart Association (AHA), the British Heart Foundation (BHF), and the Heart Foundation (Australia), offer educational resources, community programs, helplines, and advocacy efforts to support individuals affected by CHD.

-Educational Materials and Online Resources: Accessing reliable educational materials, websites, online forums, and mobile applications dedicated to CHD provides valuable information, practical tips, and resources for self-management and decision-making.

By embracing coping strategies, accessing support resources, and actively engaging in self-care practices, individuals living with CHD can enhance their quality of life, manage their condition effectively, and achieve better health outcomes over time. Regular communication with healthcare providers, ongoing education, and a proactive approach to health and wellness are vital components of successful CHD management.

Conclusion

Living with coronary heart disease (CHD) demands a comprehensive approach that encompasses various facets of cardiovascular health. Throughout the journey of managing CHD, individuals encounter pivotal strategies and resources aimed at enhancing their well-being and mitigating risks associated with the condition.

Fundamentally, lifestyle modifications serve as cornerstones in CHD management. Embracing a heart-healthy diet, engaging in regular physical activity, quitting smoking, managing stress, and maintaining a healthy weight are paramount. These lifestyle changes not only reduce the progression of CHD but also contribute to overall cardiovascular health and well-being.

In parallel, effective management of risk factors emerges as a crucial component in the prevention and treatment of CHD. Controlling blood pressure, managing lipid levels, optimizing glycemic control, and addressing comorbidities such as obesity and diabetes are essential considerations. By adhering to prescribed medications, individuals can mitigate the impact of CHD and enhance their quality of life.

Furthermore, the incorporation of coping strategies proves instrumental in navigating the challenges associated with CHD. Educating oneself about the condition, adhering to treatment plans, managing stress, and seeking social support foster resilience and empowerment. Additionally, accessing support resources such as cardiac rehabilitation programs, support groups, and patient advocacy organizations offers invaluable assistance in managing CHD and fostering a sense of community among individuals facing similar challenges.

In conclusion, empowering patients to take control of their heart health requires a collaborative effort between healthcare providers, patients, families, and communities. By embracing lifestyle modifications, adhering to treatment plans, seeking support, and staying informed, individuals can navigate the complexities of CHD management and lead fulfilling lives despite the obstacles posed by the condition. Through a holistic approach that prioritizes education, support, and proactive self-management, individuals can embark on a journey toward improved cardiovascular health and enhanced well-being in their lives.

Note

www.ingramcontent.com/pod-product-compliance
Lightning Source LLC
Chambersburg PA
CBHW070814260726
48660CB00005B/1844